Conquering Back and Sciatica Pain

Your Ultimate Guide to Relief and Restored Quality of Life

Carissa Mertz

Table of Contents

Introduction

Living with back and sciatica pain can be an overwhelming and debilitating experience, impacting every facet of your daily life. The constant discomfort, the struggle to find a comfortable position, the limitations on your physical activities, and the emotional toll can create a cycle of pain and frustration. This book, "Conquering Back and Sciatica Pain: Your Ultimate Guide to Relief and Restored Quality of Life," aims to provide you with comprehensive, practical, and effective strategies to alleviate your pain and improve your overall quality of life.

Understanding back and sciatica pain is the first step toward managing it. These conditions are often complex and multifaceted, with various causes ranging from herniated discs to spinal stenosis, muscle strain, and even psychological stress. Each individual's experience with pain is unique, requiring a personalized approach to diagnosis and treatment. In this guide, we will explore the underlying causes and symptoms of back and sciatica pain, helping you gain a clearer understanding of your condition.

Accurate diagnosis is crucial for effective treatment. This book will guide you through the medical tests and evaluations that healthcare professionals use to pinpoint the source of your pain. From physical examinations to imaging tests like MRI and CT scans, understanding these diagnostic tools will empower you to make informed decisions about your healthcare.

Treatment options for back and sciatica pain are varied, and what works for one person may not work for another. We will delve into conventional treatments, including medications and injections that can provide relief. However, medication is just one piece of the puzzle. Physical therapy plays a significant role in pain management, and we will cover a range of exercises and techniques designed to strengthen your back, improve flexibility, and reduce pain.

In addition to conventional treatments, many people find relief through alternative therapies. Acupuncture, chiropractic care, massage therapy, and other complementary approaches can offer significant benefits. This book will explore these options, providing you with a holistic view of pain management.

Nutrition and lifestyle adjustments are often overlooked but are essential components of managing back and sciatica pain. Proper nutrition supports spinal health, while lifestyle changes, such as improving your posture and ergonomics, can prevent further injury and pain. We will discuss the role of diet, supplements, and daily habits in maintaining a healthy spine.

The mind-body connection is another critical aspect of pain management. Stress and mental health can significantly impact your perception of pain and your ability to cope with it. This guide will provide strategies for stress management and improving your mental wellness, helping you build resilience against pain.

In some cases, surgical options may be necessary. Understanding when surgery is appropriate and what to expect can alleviate some of the anxiety associated with this decision. We will cover the different types of surgical interventions available, along with their risks and benefits.

Finally, this book will offer long-term strategies for maintaining a pain-free life. Pain management is not just about immediate relief; it's about building a sustainable approach to health and wellness that allows you to enjoy life to the fullest.

Whether you are at the beginning of your journey with back and sciatica pain or have been struggling for years, this comprehensive guide is designed to provide you with the knowledge, tools, and support you need to conquer your pain and restore your quality of life.

Chapter One

Understanding Back and Sciatica Pain: Causes and Symptoms

Back pain and sciatica are among the most common medical conditions that affect people worldwide. To effectively manage and alleviate this pain, it's essential to understand the underlying causes and recognize the symptoms that accompany these conditions. This chapter will provide a comprehensive overview of the causes and symptoms of back and sciatica pain, setting the stage for the various treatment strategies discussed in the subsequent chapters.

The Anatomy of the Back and Spine

The human spine is a complex structure composed of bones, muscles, ligaments, and nerves. It provides structural support, enables movement, and protects the spinal cord, a crucial part of the central nervous system. The spine is divided into several regions: cervical (neck), thoracic (mid-back), lumbar (lower back), sacral, and coccygeal (tailbone). Each region has specific functions and vulnerabilities.

The vertebrae, or spinal bones, are separated by intervertebral discs, which act as shock absorbers and allow flexibility. These discs have a tough outer layer

(called the annulus fibrosus) and a gel-like inner core (the nucleus pulposus). Surrounding the spine are muscles and ligaments that provide additional support and stability.

Common Causes of Back Pain

Back pain can arise from a variety of sources. Understanding these causes can help in diagnosing and treating the pain effectively.

Muscle Strain and Ligament Sprain: Overexertion, heavy lifting, or sudden awkward movements can cause muscles and ligaments in the back to stretch or tear. This often results in acute pain that can be severe but typically resolves with rest and conservative treatment.

Herniated or Bulging Discs: When the inner core of a spinal disc protrudes through its outer layer, it can press on nearby nerves, causing pain, numbness, or weakness. Herniated discs are common in the lumbar region due to their weight-bearing role and flexibility.

Degenerative Disc Disease: As we age, the intervertebral discs lose their water content and elasticity, leading to disc degeneration. This condition can cause chronic back pain and stiffness.

Spinal Stenosis: Narrowing of the spinal canal can put pressure on the spinal cord and nerves, leading to pain, numbness, and weakness, particularly in the legs. This condition often results from degenerative changes in the spine.

Spondylolisthesis: This occurs when a vertebra slips out of place onto the vertebra below it, causing instability and pain. It can result from degenerative changes, trauma, or congenital defects.

Osteoarthritis: The breakdown of cartilage in the joints of the spine can lead to pain, inflammation, and reduced mobility. Osteoarthritis is common in older adults and can affect any region of the spine.

Injuries and Trauma: Accidents, falls, and sports injuries can cause fractures, dislocations, and other damage to the spine and its supporting structures, leading to acute or chronic pain.

Other Medical Conditions: Conditions such as osteoporosis, scoliosis, and infections can also cause back pain. Additionally, referred pain from organs such as the kidneys or pancreas can manifest as back pain.

Understanding Sciatica

Sciatica refers to pain that radiates along the path of the sciatic nerve, which runs from the lower back through the hips and buttocks and down each leg. Sciatica typically affects only one side of the body.

Causes of Sciatica: The most common cause of sciatica is a herniated disc that presses on the sciatic nerve. Other causes include spinal stenosis, spondylolisthesis, piriformis syndrome (where the piriformis muscle compresses the sciatic nerve), and trauma.

Symptoms of Sciatica: Sciatica is characterized by pain that radiates from the lower back to the buttock and down the back of the leg. This pain can vary in intensity from a mild ache to a sharp, burning sensation. Other symptoms may include numbness, tingling, and muscle weakness in the affected leg.

Identifying Symptoms of Back and Sciatica Pain

Recognizing the symptoms of back and sciatica pain is crucial for diagnosis and treatment.

Localized Pain: Back pain can be localized to a specific area or radiate to other parts of the body. It can be dull, sharp, throbbing, or burning.

Radicular Pain: This type of pain radiates from the spine to other areas, such as the legs in sciatica. It follows the path of a nerve and can be accompanied by numbness, tingling, or weakness.

Muscle Spasms: Involuntary muscle contractions can cause severe pain and limit mobility. Muscle spasms are often a protective response to injury or inflammation.

Stiffness and Reduced Range of Motion: Pain and inflammation can lead to stiffness, making it difficult to move or perform daily activities.

Pain that Worsens with Activity: Certain movements, such as bending, lifting, or twisting, can exacerbate back pain. Conversely, rest may alleviate the pain.

Pain that Improves with Rest: Acute back pain often improves with rest and avoidance of activities that trigger the pain. However, prolonged inactivity can also lead to stiffness and weakness.

When to Seek Medical Attention

While many cases of back and sciatica pain improve with self-care and conservative treatment, certain symptoms warrant immediate medical attention:

- Severe or persistent pain that does not improve with rest or treatment
- Pain following a traumatic injury, such as a fall or accident
- Pain accompanied by fever, unexplained weight loss, or other signs of infection
- Weakness, numbness, or tingling in the legs or groin area
- Loss of bladder or bowel control, which may indicate cauda equina syndrome, a medical emergency

Chapter Two

Diagnosing Your Pain: Medical Tests and Evaluations

Accurate diagnosis is crucial for effective treatment of back and sciatica pain. This chapter will guide you through the various medical tests and evaluations that healthcare professionals use to pinpoint the source of your pain. Understanding these diagnostic tools will empower you to make informed decisions about your healthcare.

Initial Evaluation and Medical History

The first step in diagnosing back and sciatica pain is a thorough medical evaluation. Your healthcare provider will begin by taking a detailed medical history and conducting a physical examination.

<u>Medical History:</u> You will be asked about your symptoms, including the nature, location, and duration of your pain. Your doctor will also inquire about any previous injuries, medical conditions, and family history of spine-related issues. Information about your lifestyle, occupation, and activities can provide valuable insights into potential causes of your pain.

<u>Physical Examination:</u> During the physical exam, your doctor will assess your posture, range of motion, and physical condition. They will palpate (feel) your spine, muscles, and joints to identify tender areas, muscle spasms, or abnormalities. Specific tests may be performed to evaluate your nerve function and identify the presence of sciatica.

- *Range of Motion Tests:* These tests assess your ability to move your spine in various directions. Restricted or painful movements can indicate specific conditions affecting the spine.
- *Straight Leg Raise Test:* This test involves lying on your back while the doctor raises one of your legs. If this maneuver reproduces your sciatic pain, it suggests nerve root irritation or compression.

- ***Neurological Examination:*** This includes testing your reflexes, muscle strength, and sensory perception. Abnormal findings can help localize the source of nerve involvement.

Imaging Studies

Imaging studies provide a detailed view of the spine's structure, helping to identify abnormalities that may be causing your pain. Common imaging tests include:

X-Rays: X-rays are typically the first imaging test ordered for back pain. They can reveal fractures, alignment issues, and degenerative changes in the spine, such as osteoarthritis or spondylolisthesis. However, X-rays do not provide detailed information about soft tissues like discs, muscles, or nerves.

Magnetic Resonance Imaging (MRI): MRI is a powerful imaging tool that uses magnetic fields and radio waves to produce detailed images of the spine's soft tissues. It is particularly useful for diagnosing herniated discs, spinal stenosis, and other conditions affecting the spinal cord and nerve roots. MRI can also detect tumors, infections, and inflammatory processes.

Computed Tomography (CT) Scan: CT scans combine X-ray images taken from different angles to create cross-sectional views of the spine. They provide more detailed information than standard X-rays and are useful for evaluating complex fractures, bone abnormalities, and certain soft tissue conditions. CT myelography, which involves injecting a contrast dye into the spinal canal, can enhance the visibility of spinal structures.

Bone Scans: A bone scan involves injecting a small amount of radioactive material into your bloodstream. This material collects in areas of high bone activity, which can indicate fractures, infections, tumors, or other bone disorders. Bone scans are less commonly used but can be helpful in specific situations.

Electromyography (EMG) and Nerve Conduction Studies (NCS)

EMG and NCS are tests that evaluate the electrical activity of muscles and nerves. They can help determine the extent of nerve damage and identify specific nerves involved in your pain.

Electromyography (EMG): During an EMG, small needles are inserted into muscles to measure their electrical activity at rest and during contraction. Abnormal activity can indicate nerve or muscle damage.

Nerve Conduction Studies (NCS): NCS involves placing electrodes on the skin overlying a nerve and applying a small electrical stimulus. The speed and strength of the nerve's response are measured to assess nerve function. This test can identify nerve compression or damage.

Other Diagnostic Procedures

In some cases, additional diagnostic procedures may be necessary to obtain a comprehensive understanding of your condition.

Discography: Discography involves injecting a contrast dye into the intervertebral discs under X-ray guidance. The dye helps outline the disc structure, and the procedure can identify discs that are causing pain. This test is typically reserved for cases where surgery is being considered.

Facet Joint Injections: Facet joints are small joints between the vertebrae that can become inflamed and painful. Injections of anesthetic and steroid medication into these joints can help diagnose and treat facet joint pain.

Epidural Steroid Injections: An epidural injection delivers steroid medication directly into the epidural space around the spinal cord and nerve roots. This can reduce inflammation and pain, providing both diagnostic and therapeutic benefits.

Differential Diagnosis

Back and sciatica pain can result from various conditions, some of which may present with similar symptoms. A differential diagnosis involves considering multiple potential causes and systematically ruling them out through clinical evaluation and diagnostic testing.

Mechanical Back Pain: Conditions like muscle strain, ligament sprain, and degenerative disc disease fall under this category. These conditions are often related to physical activity and posture.

Radiculopathy: This refers to nerve root compression, often caused by herniated discs or spinal stenosis. Symptoms include radiating pain, numbness, and weakness.

Inflammatory Conditions: Conditions such as ankylosing spondylitis or other forms of arthritis can cause chronic back pain and stiffness, particularly in the morning.

<u>**Infections:**</u> Spinal infections, such as osteomyelitis or discitis, can cause severe pain, fever, and other systemic symptoms. These conditions require prompt medical attention.

<u>**Tumors:**</u> Spinal tumors, whether benign or malignant, can cause pain and neurological symptoms due to compression of spinal structures. Imaging studies are essential for diagnosis.

<u>**Visceral Pain:**</u> Pain originating from internal organs, such as the kidneys, pancreas, or gastrointestinal tract, can sometimes be referred to as the back. A thorough medical evaluation is necessary to identify these cases.

Collaboration with Specialists

In complex cases or when initial treatments are not effective, collaboration with specialists such as neurologists, rheumatologists, pain management specialists, and orthopedic or neurosurgeons may be necessary. These experts can provide additional insights, advanced diagnostic testing, and specialized treatments.

Chapter Three

Conventional Treatments: Medications and Injections

Once an accurate diagnosis has been made, the next step in managing back and sciatica pain is determining the appropriate treatment plan. Conventional treatments, including medications and injections, play a crucial role in alleviating pain, reducing inflammation, and improving overall function. This chapter will provide an in-depth look at the various conventional treatment options available, helping you understand their uses, benefits, and potential side effects.

Medications

Medications are often the first line of treatment for back and sciatica pain. They can provide significant relief and help manage symptoms while other therapies are implemented.

Over-the-Counter Pain Relievers: These medications are readily available without a prescription and can be effective for mild to moderate pain.

- ***Nonsteroidal Anti-Inflammatory Drugs (NSAIDs):*** Examples include ibuprofen (Advil, Motrin) and naproxen (Aleve). NSAIDs work by reducing inflammation, which helps alleviate pain and swelling. Common side effects include gastrointestinal issues, such as stomach pain, ulcers, and bleeding, especially with long-term use.

- ***Acetaminophen (Tylenol):*** This medication helps reduce pain but does not have anti-inflammatory properties. It is generally well-tolerated, but high doses can cause liver damage.

<u>Prescription Medications:</u> For more severe pain, your doctor may prescribe stronger medications.

- ***Muscle Relaxants:*** Drugs such as cyclobenzaprine (Flexeril) and methocarbamol (Robaxin) can help relieve muscle spasms associated with back pain. Side effects may include drowsiness, dizziness, and dry mouth.

- ***Opioids:*** Medications like oxycodone (OxyContin) and hydrocodone (Vicodin) are prescribed for short-term use in cases of severe pain. Due to the risk of addiction and other serious side effects, opioids are generally reserved for acute pain or flare-ups.

- ***Anticonvulsants:*** Medications such as gabapentin (Neurontin) and pregabalin (Lyrica) are used to treat nerve-related pain, including sciatica. These drugs can cause side effects like dizziness, drowsiness, and weight gain.

- ***Antidepressants:*** Certain antidepressants, such as amitriptyline and duloxetine (Cymbalta), are effective in managing chronic pain by altering the way the brain perceives pain. They can also help with sleep disturbances and mood disorders. Potential side effects include dry mouth, weight gain, and fatigue.

<u>**Topical Treatments:**</u> Creams, gels, and patches applied to the skin can provide localized pain relief.

- ***Topical NSAIDs:*** These products, such as diclofenac gel (Voltaren), can reduce pain and inflammation with fewer systemic side effects compared to oral NSAIDs.
- ***Capsaicin Cream:*** Derived from chili peppers, capsaicin cream can reduce pain by depleting a neurotransmitter involved in pain perception. Some people experience a burning sensation when first applying the cream.
- ***Lidocaine Patches:*** These patches provide localized numbness and can be particularly useful for nerve pain.

Injections

Injections deliver medication directly to the source of pain and inflammation, providing more targeted relief. They are often used when oral medications are not effective or suitable.

Epidural Steroid Injections: These injections deliver a corticosteroid, such as methylprednisolone, into the epidural space around the spinal cord and nerve roots. The steroid reduces inflammation and can provide significant pain relief for conditions like herniated discs and spinal stenosis.

- **Procedure:** The injection is usually performed under fluoroscopic (X-ray) guidance to ensure accurate placement. A local anesthetic may be used to numb the area before the injection.
- **Benefits:** Epidural steroid injections can provide relief for several weeks to months, allowing patients to participate more fully in physical therapy and other rehabilitative treatments.
- **Risks and Side Effects:** Potential risks include infection, bleeding, and nerve damage. Some patients may experience temporary increases in pain, headaches, or side effects from the steroid, such as increased blood sugar levels.

Facet Joint Injections: Facet joints are small joints between the vertebrae that can become inflamed and painful. Injections of a corticosteroid and local anesthetic into these joints can help reduce pain and inflammation.

- ***Procedure:*** Similar to epidural injections, facet joint injections are typically performed under imaging guidance. The doctor will use a needle to inject the medication directly into the affected joint.
- ***Benefits:*** Pain relief from facet joint injections can last from weeks to months, allowing patients to engage in physical therapy and other activities that promote long-term recovery.
- ***Risks and Side Effects:*** Risks include infection, bleeding, and allergic reactions. Some patients may experience temporary increases in pain or side effects from the steroid.

<u>**Nerve Blocks:**</u> Nerve blocks involve injecting an anesthetic and corticosteroid near specific nerves to block pain signals.

- ***Procedure:*** Depending on the location of the pain, different types of nerve blocks may be used, such as a selective nerve root block for sciatica. Imaging guidance is often used to ensure accurate placement.

- **Benefits:** Nerve blocks can provide immediate pain relief and help identify the specific nerve causing the pain. This can be particularly useful for diagnostic purposes.

- **Risks and Side Effects:** Risks include infection, bleeding, and nerve damage. Side effects may include temporary numbness or weakness in the affected area.

<u>**Trigger Point Injections:**</u> Trigger points are tight, painful areas of muscle that can cause referred pain. Injections of a local anesthetic and corticosteroid into these points can help alleviate pain.

- **Procedure:** The doctor will use a small needle to inject the medication directly into the trigger point. Multiple trigger points can be treated in one session.

- ***Benefits:*** Trigger point injections can provide immediate relief and help reduce muscle spasms and referred pain.

- ***Risks and Side Effects:*** Risks include infection, bleeding, and temporary soreness at the injection site.

Combination Therapies

In many cases, a combination of medications and injections is used to manage back and sciatica pain. This multimodal approach can provide more comprehensive relief and improve overall function.

- ***Medication and Physical Therapy:*** Combining medications with physical therapy can enhance the effectiveness of both treatments. Medications can reduce pain and inflammation, making it easier to participate in physical therapy exercises that strengthen the back and improve flexibility.

- ***Injections and Rehabilitation:*** Injections can provide significant pain relief, allowing patients to engage more fully in rehabilitation programs. This can lead to better long-term outcomes by addressing the underlying causes of pain.

- ***Multidisciplinary Approach:*** For chronic or severe pain, a multidisciplinary approach involving pain management specialists, physical therapists, and other healthcare providers can be beneficial. This comprehensive approach addresses the physical, emotional, and psychological aspects of pain.

Chapter Four

Physical Therapy: Exercises and Techniques for Pain Relief

Physical therapy is a cornerstone of treatment for back and sciatica pain. It focuses on improving strength, flexibility, and function while reducing pain. A well-designed physical therapy program can help prevent future episodes of pain and enhance overall quality of life. This chapter will explore various physical therapy exercises and techniques that can effectively relieve back and sciatica pain.

The Role of Physical Therapy in Pain Management

Physical therapy aims to address the underlying causes of back and sciatica pain by improving the mechanical function of the spine and its supporting structures. A physical therapist will create a personalized program based on your specific condition, symptoms, and fitness level. The primary goals of physical therapy include:

- Reducing pain and inflammation

- Improving mobility and flexibility
- Strengthening muscles that support the spine
- Enhancing posture and body mechanics
- Preventing the recurrence of pain

Core Strengthening Exercises

The core muscles, including the abdominals, back muscles, and pelvic floor, play a crucial role in supporting the spine. Strengthening these muscles can alleviate stress on the back and reduce pain.

Pelvic Tilts

- *How to Perform:* Lie on your back with your knees bent and feet flat on the floor. Tighten your abdominal muscles and flatten your lower back against the floor. Hold for a few seconds, then relax. Repeat 10-15 times.
- *Benefits:* Pelvic tilts strengthen the lower abdominal muscles and improve pelvic stability.

<u>**Bridges**</u>

- ***How to Perform:*** Lie on your back with your knees bent and feet flat on the floor. Tighten your abdominal muscles and lift your hips off the floor until your body forms a straight line from your shoulders to your knees. Hold for a few seconds, then lower your hips back to the floor. Repeat 10-15 times.
- ***Benefits:*** Bridges strengthen the gluteal muscles, hamstrings, and lower back muscles.

<u>**Planks**</u>

- ***How to Perform:*** Lie face down on the floor, then raise your body onto your forearms and toes, keeping your body in a straight line from head to heels. Hold for 20-30 seconds, gradually increasing the duration as you build strength.
- ***Benefits:*** Planks engage the entire core, including the abdominals, back muscles, and shoulders.

<u>**Bird-Dog Exercise**</u>

How to Perform: Start on your hands and knees with your wrists under your shoulders and your knees under your hips. Extend your right arm forward and your left leg backwards simultaneously, keeping your back flat. Hold for a few seconds, then return to the starting position. Repeat on the opposite side. Perform 10-15 repetitions on each side.

Benefits: This exercise improves balance and strengthens the core and lower back muscles.

Stretching Exercises

Stretching helps improve flexibility, reduce muscle tension, and enhance range of motion. Regular stretching can alleviate pain and prevent stiffness.

<u>**Cat-Cow Stretch**</u>

- *How to Perform:* Start on your hands and knees with your wrists under your shoulders and your knees under your hips. Inhale and arch your back, lifting your head and tailbone towards the ceiling (Cow Pose). Exhale and round your back, tucking your chin and tailbone (Cat Pose). Repeat 10-15 times.

- **Benefits:** This stretch increases flexibility in the spine and relieves tension in the back muscles.

Child's Pose

- **How to Perform:** Kneel on the floor with your big toes touching and your knees spread apart. Sit back on your heels and extend your arms forward, lowering your chest towards the floor. Hold for 20-30 seconds.
- **Benefits:** Child's Pose gently stretches the lower back, hips, and thighs.

Hamstring Stretch

- **How to Perform:** Lie on your back with one leg extended on the floor. Lift the other leg towards the ceiling, holding the back of your thigh with both hands. Keep your knee slightly bent. Hold for 20-30 seconds, then switch legs.

- *Benefits:* Stretching the hamstrings can reduce tension in the lower back and improve flexibility.

Piriformis Stretch

- *How to Perform:* Lie on your back with your knees bent and feet flat on the floor. Cross your right ankle over your left knee, forming a figure-four shape. Gently pull your left thigh towards your chest, holding the stretch for 20-30 seconds. Switch sides and repeat.
- *Benefits:* This stretch targets the piriformis muscle, which can relieve sciatica pain caused by piriformis syndrome.

Aerobic Exercises

Aerobic exercises, such as walking, swimming, and cycling, increase blood flow, promote healing, and improve overall fitness. Low-impact aerobic activities are particularly beneficial for individuals with back pain.

Walking

- ***How to Perform:*** Start with a brisk walk for 10-15 minutes, gradually increasing the duration as your fitness improves. Aim for 30 minutes of walking most days of the week.
- ***Benefits:*** Walking strengthens the back and leg muscles, improves cardiovascular health, and promotes weight loss, which can reduce stress on the spine.

Swimming

- ***How to Perform:*** Engage in swimming or water aerobics exercises. The buoyancy of water reduces stress on the spine while providing resistance for muscle strengthening.
- ***Benefits:*** Swimming improves overall muscle strength, flexibility, and cardiovascular fitness without placing undue strain on the back.

<u>**Cycling**</u>

- ***How to Perform:*** Use a stationary bike or ride a bicycle on flat terrain. Start with short sessions, gradually increasing the duration and intensity.
- ***Benefits:*** Cycling strengthens the lower body muscles and improves cardiovascular health. Ensure proper bike fit to avoid additional strain on the back.

Manual Therapy Techniques

Manual therapy involves hands-on techniques performed by a physical therapist to mobilize joints, reduce pain, and improve function.

<u>**Spinal Mobilization**</u>

- ***How it Works:*** The therapist uses gentle, passive movements to improve joint mobility and reduce pain. This technique is often used for patients with limited range of motion or stiffness.

- ***Benefits:*** Spinal mobilization can relieve pain, improve flexibility, and enhance overall function.

Soft Tissue Mobilization

- ***How it Works:*** The therapist applies pressure to the muscles and soft tissues to reduce tension, improve circulation, and promote healing.
- ***Benefits:*** Soft tissue mobilization can alleviate muscle spasms, reduce pain, and improve flexibility.

Myofascial Release

- ***How it Works:*** The therapist uses sustained pressure to release tension in the fascia, the connective tissue surrounding muscles and organs.
- ***Benefits:*** Myofascial release can reduce pain, improve mobility, and enhance overall function.

Education and Posture Training

Proper posture and body mechanics are essential for preventing and managing back and sciatica pain. Physical therapists provide education and training to help you maintain good posture and avoid movements that exacerbate pain.

Ergonomic Training

- *How it Works:* The therapist assesses your work environment and daily activities, providing recommendations for ergonomic adjustments. This may include proper desk setup, lifting techniques, and standing or sitting posture.
- *Benefits:* Ergonomic training can reduce stress on the spine, prevent injury, and alleviate pain.

Posture Correction Exercises

- *How to Perform:* Exercises such as scapular retractions, chin tucks, and wall angels can improve posture and strengthen the muscles that support proper alignment.

- ***Benefits:*** Good posture reduces strain on the spine, alleviates pain, and prevents future episodes of back pain.

Chapter Five

Exploring Holistic and Complementary Treatments

While conventional treatments and physical therapy are fundamental in managing back and sciatica pain, many people find additional relief through alternative and complementary therapies. These holistic approaches can enhance conventional treatments, offering a more comprehensive and personalized pain management plan. This chapter explores various alternative therapies that have shown promise in alleviating back and sciatica pain.

Acupuncture

Acupuncture, a key component of traditional Chinese medicine, involves inserting thin needles into specific points on the body to balance the flow of energy (Qi). It has gained popularity as a treatment for chronic pain, including back and sciatica pain.

How Acupuncture Works

- **Theory:** According to traditional Chinese medicine, pain is caused by blocked or imbalanced Qi flow. Acupuncture aims to restore balance and promote healing.
- **Scientific Perspective:** Modern research suggests that acupuncture may stimulate the release of endorphins, the body's natural painkillers, and affect the nervous system, reducing pain perception.

Procedure

- **Initial Consultation:** The acupuncturist will take a detailed medical history and assess your condition to determine the appropriate acupuncture points.
- **Treatment Session:** Thin, sterile needles are inserted into specific points and left in place for 20-40 minutes. You may feel a slight tingling or warmth at the needle sites.

Benefits

- ***Pain Relief:*** Many studies have shown that acupuncture can reduce pain and improve function in individuals with chronic back pain and sciatica.

- ***Overall Well-being:*** Acupuncture can promote relaxation, reduce stress, and improve overall well-being.

Risks and Considerations

- ***Safety:*** Acupuncture is generally safe when performed by a licensed practitioner. However, potential risks include infection, bruising, and minor bleeding.

- ***Contraindications:*** Certain conditions, such as bleeding disorders or pregnancy, may require special precautions.

Chiropractic Care

Chiropractic care focuses on diagnosing and treating musculoskeletal disorders, particularly those involving the spine. Chiropractors use hands-on spinal manipulation and other techniques to improve alignment and relieve pain.

Spinal Manipulation

- *How it Works:* The chiropractor applies controlled, sudden force to a spinal joint, aiming to improve spinal motion and reduce pain.

- *Benefits:* Spinal manipulation can provide immediate pain relief, improve function, and enhance overall mobility.

Additional Techniques

- *Mobilization:* Gentle, slow movements of the joints to improve range of motion.

- *Soft Tissue Therapy:* Techniques such as massage and myofascial release to reduce muscle tension and improve circulation.

- *Exercise and Lifestyle Counseling:* Chiropractors often provide guidance on exercises, posture, and lifestyle modifications to support long-term health.

<u>**Risks and Considerations**</u>

- ***Safety:*** Chiropractic care is generally safe when performed by a licensed practitioner. Potential risks include temporary discomfort, headaches, and, in rare cases, serious complications such as stroke.
- ***Contraindications:*** Individuals with certain medical conditions, such as severe osteoporosis or spinal instability, may need to avoid spinal manipulation.

Massage Therapy

Massage therapy involves manipulating the soft tissues of the body, including muscles, connective tissues, and tendons, to relieve pain and promote healing. Different types of massage can benefit individuals with back and sciatica pain.

<u>**Types of Massage**</u>

- ***Swedish Massage:*** Uses long, gliding strokes, kneading, and circular movements to relax and energize the body.

- ***Deep Tissue Massage:*** Focuses on the deeper layers of muscle and connective tissue, using slower, more forceful strokes to relieve chronic pain and muscle tension.
- ***Trigger Point Therapy:*** Targets specific trigger points or knots in the muscles that can refer pain to other areas of the body.

Benefits

- ***Pain Relief:*** Massage can reduce muscle tension, improve circulation, and decrease inflammation, leading to pain relief.
- ***Relaxation and Stress Reduction:*** Massage promotes relaxation, reduces stress, and improves overall well-being.

Risks and Considerations

- ***Safety:*** Massage therapy is generally safe when performed by a trained therapist. Potential risks include temporary soreness, bruising, and, in rare cases, nerve damage.

- *Contraindications:* Certain medical conditions, such as blood clotting disorders or infections, may require special precautions.

Yoga and Pilates

Yoga and Pilates are mind-body practices that focus on strengthening the body, improving flexibility, and enhancing overall well-being. Both practices can be beneficial for individuals with back and sciatica pain.

<u>Yoga</u>

- *How it Works:* Yoga combines physical postures, breathing exercises, and meditation to promote physical and mental health.
- *Benefits:* Yoga can improve flexibility, strength, and posture, reduce stress, and alleviate pain. Specific yoga poses, such as Child's Pose and Cat-Cow Stretch, can target the back and relieve tension.

Pilates

- *How it Works:* Pilates focuses on strengthening the core muscles, improving posture, and enhancing overall body alignment.
- *Benefits:* Pilates exercises, such as the Hundred and Pelvic Tilts, can strengthen the muscles that support the spine, reduce pain, and improve function.

Risks and Considerations

- *Safety:* Both yoga and Pilates are generally safe when performed correctly. However, improper technique or pushing beyond one's limits can lead to injury.
- *Contraindications:* Certain conditions, such as severe osteoporosis or acute injuries, may require modifications or avoidance of specific poses or exercises.

Herbal and Nutritional Supplements

Certain herbal and nutritional supplements have been used to manage pain and inflammation. While research on their efficacy is ongoing, some supplements have shown promise in relieving back and sciatica pain.

Common Supplements

- **Turmeric:** Contains curcumin, a compound with anti-inflammatory properties. Turmeric supplements may help reduce inflammation and pain.
- **Devil's Claw:** An herb traditionally used for pain and inflammation. Some studies suggest it may be effective in reducing back pain.
- **Omega-3 Fatty Acids:** Found in fish oil, these fatty acids have anti-inflammatory properties and may help reduce pain.

<u>**Benefits**</u>

- ***Pain and Inflammation Reduction:*** Some supplements may help reduce pain and inflammation, improving overall function.
- ***Overall Health:*** Nutritional supplements can support overall health and well-being.

<u>**Risks and Considerations**</u>

- ***Safety:*** While many supplements are generally safe, potential risks include interactions with medications, allergic reactions, and side effects. It is essential to consult a healthcare provider before starting any new supplement.
- ***Quality and Efficacy:*** The quality and efficacy of supplements can vary. Choosing high-quality products from reputable sources is important.

Mind-Body Techniques

Mind-body techniques focus on the connection between the mind and body, using mental and emotional practices to influence physical health and manage pain.

Meditation and Mindfulness

- *How it Works:* Meditation and mindfulness practices involve focusing the mind, calming the nervous system, and promoting relaxation.
- *Benefits:* These practices can reduce stress, improve pain tolerance, and enhance overall well-being.

Biofeedback

- *How it Works:* Biofeedback involves using electronic devices to monitor physiological functions, such as heart rate and muscle tension. By becoming aware of these functions, individuals can learn to control them and reduce pain.
- *Benefits:* Biofeedback can help manage chronic pain, reduce stress, and improve overall health.

Cognitive-Behavioral Therapy (CBT)

- *How it Works:* CBT is a form of psychotherapy that focuses on changing negative thought patterns and behaviors. It can help individuals develop coping strategies for managing pain.
- *Benefits:* CBT can reduce pain, improve mood, and enhance overall quality of life.

Chapter Six

The Role of Nutrition in Managing Pain

Nutrition plays a significant role in overall health, including the management of back and sciatica pain. The foods you eat can influence inflammation, muscle health, and pain perception. This chapter explores the importance of a balanced diet, specific nutrients that can help reduce pain and inflammation, and dietary strategies to support spine health and overall well-being.

Understanding the Link Between Diet and Pain

The connection between diet and pain is multifaceted. Certain foods can promote inflammation and exacerbate pain, while others can reduce inflammation and support the body's healing processes. A diet rich in anti-inflammatory foods and essential nutrients can help manage chronic pain and improve overall health.

Anti-Inflammatory Diet

An anti-inflammatory diet focuses on foods that reduce inflammation and support the body's natural healing processes. Chronic inflammation is a common contributor to back and sciatica pain, and reducing it can alleviate symptoms and improve function.

Fruits and Vegetables

- *Benefits:* Fruits and vegetables are rich in antioxidants, vitamins, and minerals that combat inflammation and support overall health.

- *Recommendations:* Aim to include a variety of colorful fruits and vegetables in your diet, such as berries, leafy greens, carrots, and tomatoes.

Whole Grains

- *Benefits:* Whole grains are high in fiber, which can reduce inflammation and support digestive health.

- *Recommendations:* Choose whole grains such as brown rice, quinoa, oats, and whole wheat bread over refined grains.

Healthy Fats

- *Benefits:* Healthy fats, particularly omega-3 fatty acids, have strong anti-inflammatory properties.
- *Recommendations:* Include sources of healthy fats in your diet, such as fatty fish (salmon, mackerel, sardines), flaxseeds, chia seeds, walnuts, and olive oil.

Lean Proteins

- *Benefits:* Lean proteins provide essential amino acids that support muscle health and repair.
- *Recommendations:* Choose lean protein sources such as chicken, turkey, tofu, legumes, and low-fat dairy products.

<u>**Herbs and Spices**</u>

- ***Benefits:*** Many herbs and spices, such as turmeric, ginger, and garlic, have anti-inflammatory properties.

- ***Recommendations:*** Incorporate a variety of herbs and spices into your meals to enhance flavor and provide health benefits.

Essential Nutrients for Spine Health

Certain nutrients play a crucial role in maintaining the health of your spine and reducing pain. Ensuring adequate intake of these nutrients can support the structural integrity and function of your spine.

<u>**Calcium**</u>

- ***Benefits:*** Calcium is essential for strong bones and teeth. It supports bone density and helps prevent osteoporosis, which can contribute to back pain.

- ***Sources:*** Dairy products (milk, cheese, yogurt), leafy green vegetables (kale, broccoli), fortified plant-based milks, and almonds.

Vitamin D

- **Benefits:** Vitamin D enhances calcium absorption and supports bone health. It also has anti-inflammatory properties.
- **Sources:** Sunlight exposure, fatty fish (salmon, mackerel), fortified dairy and plant-based milk, and egg yolks.

Magnesium

- **Benefits:** Magnesium supports muscle and nerve function and helps maintain healthy bone density. It also has anti-inflammatory properties.
- **Sources:** Leafy green vegetables, nuts and seeds, whole grains, legumes, and dark chocolate.

<u>**Vitamin C**</u>

- ***Benefits:*** Vitamin C is a powerful antioxidant that supports collagen formation, essential for the health of cartilage, ligaments, and tendons.
- ***Sources:*** Citrus fruits (oranges, grapefruits), berries, bell peppers, and broccoli.

<u>**Vitamin B12**</u>

- ***Benefits***: Vitamin B12 supports nerve health and can help reduce neuropathic pain.
- ***Sources***: Animal products (meat, fish, dairy), fortified cereals, and nutritional yeast.

Hydration and Pain Management

Staying well-hydrated is essential for overall health and can influence pain perception and muscle function. Dehydration can lead to muscle cramps and worsen pain.

<u>**Water Intake**</u>

- *Benefits*: Adequate water intake supports cellular function, aids digestion, and helps maintain muscle and joint health.
- *Recommendations*: Aim to drink at least 8 glasses (about 2 liters) of water per day, more if you are physically active or live in a hot climate.

<u>**Hydrating Foods**</u>

- *Benefits*: Consuming foods with high water content can contribute to overall hydration.
- *Recommendations*: Include hydrating foods in your diet, such as cucumbers, watermelon, oranges, and lettuce.

Foods to Avoid

Certain foods can exacerbate inflammation and pain. Limiting or avoiding these foods can help manage back and sciatica pain.

Processed Foods

- *Risks*: Processed foods often contain high levels of unhealthy fats, sugar, and sodium, which can promote inflammation.
- *Examples*: Snack foods, fast food, sugary beverages, and pre-packaged meals.

Refined Carbohydrates

- *Risks*: Refined carbohydrates can cause spikes in blood sugar levels and promote inflammation.
- *Examples*: White bread, pastries, sugary cereals, and white rice.

Saturated and Trans Fats

- *Risks*: These fats can increase inflammation and contribute to various health issues.
- *Examples*: Fried foods, baked goods with hydrogenated oils, and fatty cuts of meat.

<u>**Excessive Alcohol**</u>

- ***Risks***: Excessive alcohol consumption can increase inflammation and interfere with pain management.
- ***Recommendations***: Limit alcohol intake to moderate levels (up to one drink per day for women and up to two drinks per day for men).

Practical Dietary Strategies

Implementing a balanced diet that supports spine health and reduces inflammation involves practical strategies that can be easily integrated into daily life.

<u>**Meal Planning**</u>

- ***Benefits***: Planning meals in advance can help ensure a balanced diet and prevent reliance on unhealthy convenience foods.
- ***Tips***: Create a weekly meal plan, prepare grocery lists, and batch-cook meals to save time and effort.

Mindful Eating

- ***Benefits***: Paying attention to hunger and fullness cues can prevent overeating and support healthy weight management, reducing stress on the spine.
- ***Tips***: Eat slowly, savor each bite, and avoid distractions such as television or smartphones during meals.

Balanced Meals

- ***Benefits***: Consuming balanced meals with a mix of protein, healthy fats, fiber, and carbohydrates can support energy levels and overall health.
- ***Tips***: Aim to fill half your plate with vegetables, a quarter with lean protein, and a quarter with whole grains or healthy carbs.

<u>**Healthy Snacks**</u>

- ***Benefits***: Choosing healthy snacks can maintain energy levels and prevent overeating during meals.
- ***Tips***: Opt for snacks such as fresh fruit, nuts, yogurt, or whole-grain crackers with hummus.

Chapter Seven

Lifestyle Adjustments for Pain Management

Lifestyle factors such as physical activity, sleep quality, stress management, and ergonomics can all impact pain levels and overall well-being. This chapter explores practical lifestyle adjustments that can help reduce pain, improve function, and enhance quality of life.

Physical Activity and Exercise

Physical activity is essential for maintaining spinal health, strengthening muscles, and reducing pain. Regular exercise can improve flexibility, mobility, and posture, reducing the risk of injury and relieving back and sciatica pain.

Low-Impact Activities

- **Benefits**: Activities such as walking, swimming, and cycling are gentle on the spine and provide cardiovascular benefits without placing excessive strain on the back.

- *Recommendations*: Aim for at least 30 minutes of moderate-intensity aerobic exercise most days of the week, supplemented with strength training and flexibility exercises.

Core Strengthening

- *Benefits*: Strengthening the core muscles, including the abdominals, back muscles, and pelvic floor, provides stability and support for the spine, reducing the risk of injury and alleviating pain.
- *Exercises*: Include core-strengthening exercises such as planks, bridges, and bird-dog exercises in your exercise routine.

Flexibility and Stretching

- *Benefits*: Improving flexibility in the muscles and ligaments surrounding the spine can reduce stiffness, improve range of motion, and alleviate pain.
- *Exercises*: Incorporate stretching exercises such as yoga, Pilates, and specific stretches

targeting the back, hamstrings, and hips into your daily routine.

Sleep Hygiene

Quality sleep is essential for overall health and well-being, including pain management. Poor sleep quality can exacerbate pain, while adequate restorative sleep can reduce inflammation, improve mood, and enhance pain tolerance.

Optimal Sleep Environment

- ***Recommendations***: Create a sleep-friendly environment by ensuring your bedroom is dark, quiet, and cool. Invest in a comfortable mattress and pillows that support spinal alignment.

Consistent Sleep Schedule

- ***Recommendations***: Establish a regular sleep schedule by going to bed and waking up at the same time each day, even on weekends. Consistency helps regulate your body's internal clock and improves sleep quality.

<u>**Relaxation Techniques**</u>

- ***Benefits***: Practicing relaxation techniques such as deep breathing, meditation, or progressive muscle relaxation before bedtime can calm the mind and body, promoting restful sleep.

- ***Recommendations***: Incorporate relaxation exercises into your bedtime routine to signal to your body that it's time to wind down and prepare for sleep.

Stress Management

Chronic stress can exacerbate pain and contribute to muscle tension and inflammation. Effective stress management techniques can help reduce stress levels, alleviate pain, and improve overall well-being.

<u>**Mindfulness Meditation**</u>

- ***Benefits***: Mindfulness meditation involves focusing on the present moment without judgment, which can reduce stress, promote relaxation, and enhance pain tolerance.

- *Practices*: Dedicate time each day to mindfulness meditation, focusing on your breath, bodily sensations, or a guided meditation.

Yoga and Tai Chi

- *Benefits*: Yoga and Tai Chi combine gentle movements, deep breathing, and meditation to promote relaxation, reduce stress, and improve flexibility and balance.
- *Practices*: Attend regular yoga or Tai Chi classes or follow online videos to incorporate these practices into your routine.

Cognitive-Behavioral Therapy (CBT)

- *Benefits*: CBT helps identify and change negative thought patterns and behaviors that contribute to stress and pain. It provides practical strategies for coping with pain and improving overall quality of life.

- ***Therapy***: Consider working with a therapist trained in CBT to develop personalized coping strategies and techniques for managing stress and pain.

Ergonomics and Posture

Proper ergonomics and posture are essential for preventing and reducing back and sciatica pain, particularly for individuals who spend long hours sitting or performing repetitive tasks.

Workstation Setup

- ***Recommendations***: Adjust your workstation to promote proper posture and reduce strain on the spine. Ensure your chair provides adequate support for your lower back, and position your computer screen at eye level to prevent neck strain.

Lifting Techniques

- ***Recommendations***: Use proper lifting techniques to protect your back when lifting heavy objects. Bend at the knees, keep the object close to your body, and lift with your legs rather than your back.

Body Mechanics

- ***Recommendations***: Practice good body mechanics throughout the day, maintaining neutral spine alignment when sitting, standing, and moving. Avoid slouching or rounding your shoulders, which can strain the back muscles.

Leisure Activities and Hobbies

Engaging in leisure activities and hobbies that bring joy and fulfillment can have a positive impact on mental and emotional well-being, reducing stress and improving the overall quality of life.

Low-Impact Recreational Activities

- ***Recommendations***: Participate in low-impact recreational activities such as gardening, gentle hiking, or recreational swimming to stay active and maintain mobility without exacerbating pain.

Creative Outlets

- **Benefits**: Engaging in creative outlets such as painting, writing, or playing music can provide a sense of accomplishment, reduce stress, and distract from pain.
- **Recommendations**: Dedicate time to pursue creative activities that bring joy and fulfillment, even if only for short periods each day.

Chapter Eight

Harnessing Mental and Emotional Health for Pain Relief

The mind-body connection refers to the intricate relationship between mental and emotional states and physical health. Chronic pain, including back and sciatica pain, is influenced by various factors, including stress, anxiety, depression, and coping mechanisms. Understanding and harnessing the mind-body connection can play a significant role in managing pain and improving overall well-being. This chapter explores the impact of mental and emotional health on pain perception, strategies for managing stress and negative emotions, and techniques for promoting relaxation and resilience.

The Impact of Mental and Emotional Health on Pain Perception

Mental and emotional health can profoundly influence the experience of pain. Stress, anxiety, depression, and other psychological factors can exacerbate pain perception, increase muscle tension, and contribute to the development of chronic pain conditions.

Stress and Pain

- *Relationship*: Chronic stress can heighten pain sensitivity, trigger muscle tension, and exacerbate inflammation, leading to increased pain levels.
- *Effects*: Stress-induced muscle tension can worsen back and sciatica pain, while heightened pain perception can further increase stress levels, creating a vicious cycle.

Anxiety and Pain

- *Relationship*: Anxiety amplifies pain perception and can lead to anticipatory anxiety, fear of movement, and avoidance behaviors, all of which contribute to the persistence of pain.
- *Effects*: Anxiety-related muscle tension and hypervigilance can exacerbate physical

symptoms and interfere with relaxation and pain relief.

Depression and Pain

- ***Relationship***: Depression and chronic pain often coexist, with each condition exacerbating the other. Depression can increase pain severity, impair coping mechanisms, and reduce motivation to engage in activities that provide pain relief.
- ***Effects***: Chronic pain can contribute to feelings of hopelessness, helplessness, and social isolation, exacerbating depressive symptoms and reducing quality of life.

Strategies for Managing Stress and Negative Emotions

Effective stress management and emotional regulation techniques can help reduce pain perception, alleviate muscle tension, and improve overall well-being. By cultivating resilience and coping skills, individuals can better navigate the challenges of living with chronic pain.

Mindfulness Meditation

- **Benefits**: Mindfulness meditation cultivates present-moment awareness and nonjudgmental acceptance of thoughts and emotions, reducing stress reactivity and promoting relaxation.
- **Practices**: Regular mindfulness meditation practice can include focused breathing exercises, body scans, and mindful movement (e.g., yoga, Tai Chi).

Deep Breathing Exercises

- **Benefits**: Deep breathing exercises activate the body's relaxation response, calming the nervous system and reducing physiological arousal associated with stress and anxiety.
- **Techniques**: Practice diaphragmatic breathing, box breathing, or progressive muscle relaxation to promote relaxation and alleviate muscle tension.

Cognitive Restructuring

- ***Benefits***: Cognitive restructuring involves challenging and reframing negative thoughts and beliefs that contribute to stress, anxiety, and depression.
- ***Techniques***: Identify and challenge cognitive distortions (e.g., catastrophizing, black-and-white thinking) and replace them with more balanced and realistic perspectives.

Positive Psychology Interventions

- ***Benefits***: Positive psychology interventions focus on cultivating positive emotions, strengths, and meaning in life, promoting resilience and well-being in the face of adversity.
- ***Practices***: Engage in activities such as gratitude journaling, acts of kindness, and savoring positive experiences to foster resilience and improve mood.

Relaxation Techniques for Pain Relief

Promoting relaxation is essential for managing pain and reducing muscle tension associated with chronic stress and anxiety. Incorporating relaxation techniques into daily life can help individuals achieve a greater sense of calm and well-being.

Progressive Muscle Relaxation (PMR)

- *Benefits*: PMR involves systematically tensing and relaxing muscle groups throughout the body, promoting physical relaxation and reducing muscle tension.

- *Techniques*: Practice PMR by sequentially tensing and releasing muscle groups, starting from the feet and progressing upward to the head and neck.

Guided Imagery and Visualization

- *Benefits*: Guided imagery and visualization involve using mental imagery to evoke a sense of relaxation and well-being, reducing stress and promoting healing.

- *Techniques*: Listen to guided imagery recordings or create your mental images of peaceful, serene settings to promote relaxation and pain relief.

Aromatherapy

- *Benefits*: Aromatherapy utilizes essential oils derived from plants to promote relaxation, reduce stress, and alleviate pain.
- *Techniques*: Diffuse calming essential oils such as lavender, chamomile, or peppermint in your home or add a few drops to a warm bath to enhance relaxation and promote sleep.

Music Therapy

- *Benefits*: Music therapy involves listening to or creating music to promote relaxation, reduce stress, and improve mood.

- *Techniques*: Create personalized playlists of calming music or engage in activities such as playing a musical instrument or singing to enhance relaxation and reduce pain perception.

Cultivating Resilience and Optimism

Building resilience and maintaining a positive outlook can help individuals cope with the challenges of living with chronic pain. By fostering optimism, finding meaning in adversity, and cultivating social support, individuals can enhance their ability to adapt and thrive despite pain.

Optimism and Positive Thinking

- *Benefits*: Optimism fosters a hopeful and positive outlook, enhancing coping mechanisms, reducing stress, and promoting emotional well-being.
- *Practices*: Practice gratitude, focus on strengths and accomplishments, and

challenge negative self-talk to cultivate optimism and resilience.

Finding Meaning and Purpose

- *Benefits*: Finding meaning and purpose in life can provide a sense of direction, motivation, and resilience in the face of adversity.
- *Practices*: Identify values, goals, and activities that provide meaning and fulfillment, and strive to incorporate them into daily life despite pain-related challenges.

Social Support and connection

- *Benefits*: Social support plays a crucial role in coping with chronic pain, providing emotional validation, practical assistance, and a sense of belonging.
- *Practices*: Cultivate and maintain supportive relationships with friends, family members, healthcare providers, and support groups to reduce isolation and enhance resilience.

Chapter Nine

Integrative Approaches to Pain Management: Holistic Healing for Body and Mind

Integrative medicine combines conventional medical treatments with complementary and alternative therapies to address the physical, emotional, and spiritual aspects of health and healing. In the context of pain management, integrative approaches offer a comprehensive framework for addressing back and sciatica pain by considering the interconnectedness of body, mind, and spirit. This chapter explores various integrative modalities, including acupuncture, massage therapy, chiropractic care, mindfulness-based interventions, and energy healing, and their role in promoting holistic healing for individuals living with chronic pain.

Acupuncture and Traditional Chinese Medicine (TCM)

Acupuncture, a cornerstone of Traditional Chinese Medicine (TCM), involves the insertion of thin needles into specific points on the body to stimulate energy flow and promote healing. Acupuncture is effective in relieving back and sciatica pain by reducing inflammation, improving circulation, and releasing endorphins, the body's natural painkillers.

Theory and Practice

- ***Meridian Theory:*** According to TCM, pain and illness result from imbalances or blockages in the flow of Qi (vital energy) along meridians in the body. Acupuncture aims to restore balance and harmony to the body's energy system.

- ***Treatment Approach:*** Acupuncturists select specific acupuncture points based on individual diagnosis and treatment goals, often combining needling with other modalities such as cupping, moxibustion, or herbal therapy.

<u>**Research and Evidence**</u>

- ***Clinical Studies:*** Numerous clinical studies have demonstrated the efficacy of acupuncture in reducing back pain, and sciatica symptoms, and improving overall quality of life. Meta-analyses support its use as a complementary therapy for chronic pain management.

<u>**Safety and Considerations**</u>

- ***Safety Profile:*** Acupuncture is generally safe when performed by a licensed practitioner using sterile needles. Minor side effects such as bruising or soreness may occur but are usually temporary.

- ***Contraindications***: Acupuncture may not be suitable for individuals with bleeding disorders, pacemakers, or certain medical conditions. Consultation with a qualified practitioner is recommended.

Massage Therapy and Bodywork

Massage therapy encompasses a variety of techniques aimed at manipulating soft tissues to relieve muscle tension, reduce pain, and promote relaxation. Different massage modalities, such as Swedish massage, deep tissue massage, and myofascial release, can be beneficial for individuals with back and sciatica pain.

Benefits of Massage

- **Muscle Relaxation:** Massage therapy helps release muscle tension and reduce trigger points, alleviating pain and stiffness.
- **Improved Circulation:** Massage increases blood flow to the muscles, promoting healing and reducing inflammation.
- **Stress Reduction:** The calming effects of massage can help reduce stress, anxiety, and cortisol levels, further relieving pain.

<u>**Types of Massage**</u>

- ***Swedish Massage:*** Uses long, flowing strokes, kneading, and circular movements to promote relaxation and improve circulation.

- ***Deep Tissue Massage:*** Targets deeper layers of muscle and connective tissue to release chronic tension and break up scar tissue.

- ***Myofascial Release:*** Focuses on releasing tension in the fascia, the connective tissue that surrounds muscles and organs, to alleviate pain and improve mobility.

<u>**Integration with Other Therapies**</u>

- ***Complementary Approach:*** Massage therapy can complement other pain management strategies such as physical therapy, chiropractic care, and acupuncture, enhancing overall treatment effectiveness.

- ***Individualized Treatment:*** A skilled massage therapist will tailor the treatment to address the specific needs and preferences of each individual, considering their unique pain patterns and medical history.

Chiropractic Care and Spinal Manipulation

Chiropractic care focuses on diagnosing and treating musculoskeletal disorders, particularly those involving the spine. Chiropractors use hands-on spinal manipulation and other techniques to improve spinal alignment, reduce nerve irritation, and alleviate pain associated with back and sciatica conditions.

Spinal Adjustment Techniques

- **Spinal Manipulation:** Involves applying controlled, sudden force to spinal joints to improve alignment and restore mobility. This can reduce nerve compression and alleviate pain.
- **Mobilization:** Gentle stretching and movement of the joints to improve flexibility and reduce stiffness.

<u>**Evidence and Effectiveness**</u>

- ***Research Support:*** Spinal manipulation is effective in reducing pain and improving function in individuals with acute and chronic back pain, including sciatica.

- ***Safety Considerations:*** While spinal manipulation is generally safe when performed by a trained chiropractor, there are rare risks of adverse effects such as stroke or nerve injury. Patients with certain medical conditions may require special precautions.

Mindfulness-Based Interventions and Stress Reduction Techniques

Mindfulness-based interventions, including mindfulness meditation, yoga, and Tai Chi, focus on cultivating present-moment awareness and acceptance of one's thoughts and emotions. These practices can help individuals with chronic pain manage stress, reduce pain perception, and improve overall well-being.

Mindfulness Meditation

- ***Benefits***: Mindfulness meditation teaches individuals to observe their thoughts and sensations without judgment, reducing reactivity and promoting emotional regulation.

- ***Pain Management:*** Mindfulness meditation is effective in reducing pain intensity, improving pain-related disability, and enhancing quality of life in individuals with chronic pain conditions.

Yoga and Tai Chi

- ***Physical and Mental Benefits:*** Yoga and Tai Chi combine gentle movements, breathwork, and meditation to promote relaxation, reduce muscle tension, and improve flexibility and balance.

- ***Pain Relief:*** Regular practice of yoga or Tai Chi has been associated with reduced pain severity, improved physical function, and enhanced mood in individuals with chronic pain conditions.

Stress Reduction Techniques

- ***Breathing Exercises:*** Deep breathing exercises such as diaphragmatic breathing and box breathing can activate the body's relaxation response, reducing stress and promoting calmness.

- ***Progressive Muscle Relaxation:*** Progressive muscle relaxation involves systematically tensing and relaxing muscle groups to promote physical and mental relaxation, reducing muscle tension and pain perception.

Energy Healing Modalities

Energy healing modalities such as Reiki, Healing Touch, and Qigong focus on balancing and restoring the body's energy system to promote healing and well-being. While the mechanisms of action are not fully understood, these practices are believed to influence the flow of energy within the body and facilitate self-healing processes.

Reiki

- *Principles*: Reiki involves the channeling of universal life force energy through the practitioner's hands to the recipient, promoting relaxation, stress reduction, and healing on physical, emotional, and spiritual levels.
- *Application*: Reiki sessions typically involve light touch or hands hovering over the body in specific hand positions, with the recipient fully clothed and lying comfortably on a massage table.

Healing Touch

- *Techniques*: Healing Touch incorporates gentle touch and energy-based interventions to clear, balance, and energize the body's energy system, promoting relaxation and supporting the body's natural healing processes.

- *Application*: Healing Touch practitioners use techniques such as energetic clearing, chakra balancing, and magnetic passes to facilitate energy flow and promote holistic healing.

Qigong

- *Principles*: Qigong is a mind-body practice that integrates gentle movements, breathwork, and meditation to cultivate Qi (vital energy) flow, promote health, and enhance well-being.
- *Benefits*: Regular practice of Qigong has been associated with reduced pain, improved physical function, and enhanced quality of life in individuals with chronic pain conditions.

Integrative Pain Management Programs

Integrative pain management programs offer a comprehensive approach to addressing back and sciatica pain by combining conventional medical treatments with complementary and alternative therapies. These programs often involve interdisciplinary teams of healthcare providers, including physicians, physical therapists, acupuncturists, massage therapists, and psychologists, working collaboratively to develop individualized treatment plans.

Multimodal Approach

- *Tailored Treatment:* Integrative pain management programs tailor treatment plans to address the unique needs and preferences of each individual, incorporating a combination of evidence-based therapies to optimize pain relief and improve overall well-being.

- *Holistic Assessment:* Providers conduct comprehensive assessments to identify physical, emotional, and lifestyle factors contributing to pain, guiding the selection of appropriate interventions.

Patient Education and Empowerment

- **Self-Management Skills:** Integrative pain management programs empower patients to take an active role in their healing process by providing education and resources for self-care, stress management, and pain coping strategies.

- **Shared Decision-Making:** Patients are encouraged to collaborate with their healthcare providers in making informed decisions about their treatment goals and preferences, fostering a sense of ownership and autonomy in their healthcare journey.

Chapter Ten

Self-Care Strategies for Long-Term Pain Management

Empowering yourself is a crucial aspect of managing chronic pain, including back and sciatica pain. While healthcare providers play an essential role in providing treatment and support, individuals living with pain also have the power to take control of their well-being. This chapter explores various self-care strategies and lifestyle modifications that can empower individuals to effectively manage their pain, improve function, and enhance quality of life.

Education and Understanding

Knowledge is power when it comes to managing chronic pain. Understanding the underlying causes of back and sciatica pain, as well as learning about treatment options and self-care techniques, empowers individuals to make informed decisions about their health.

<u>**Learn About Your Condition**</u>

- ***Research***: Take the time to educate yourself about the anatomy of the spine, common causes of back pain, and the mechanisms underlying sciatica.

- ***Ask Questions:*** Don't hesitate to ask your healthcare provider questions about your condition, treatment options, and prognosis. Understanding your diagnosis and treatment plan can help alleviate anxiety and empower you to take an active role in your recovery.

<u>**Stay Informed About Treatment Options**</u>

- ***Explore Options***: Familiarize yourself with various treatment modalities, including conventional medical treatments, complementary therapies, and self-care strategies.

- ***Evidence-Based Information:*** Seek out reputable sources of information, such as medical websites, peer-reviewed journals, and trusted healthcare professionals, to stay informed about evidence-based treatment options.

Pain Management Techniques

Developing effective pain management techniques is essential for coping with chronic pain on a day-to-day basis. By incorporating self-care strategies into your daily routine, you can reduce pain intensity, improve function, and enhance overall well-being.

Mind-Body Practices

- ***Mindfulness Meditation:*** Practice mindfulness meditation to cultivate present-moment awareness and reduce stress, anxiety, and pain perception.
- ***Deep Breathing Exercises:*** Engage in deep breathing exercises to promote relaxation, calm the nervous system, and reduce muscle tension.
- ***Progressive Muscle Relaxation:*** Incorporate progressive muscle relaxation techniques

into your daily routine to release tension and alleviate pain.

Movement and Exercise

- **_Low-Impact Activities:_** Participate in low-impact exercises such as walking, swimming, or cycling to improve mobility, strengthen muscles, and reduce pain.
- **_Stretching:_** Perform gentle stretching exercises to improve flexibility, alleviate stiffness, and reduce the risk of injury.
- **_Core Strengthening:_** Focus on strengthening the core muscles to provide stability and support for the spine, reducing the risk of back pain and sciatica.

Heat and Cold Therapy

- **_Heat Therapy:_** Apply heat packs or warm towels to the affected area to increase blood flow, relax muscles, and alleviate pain and stiffness.

- ***Cold Therapy:*** Use ice packs or cold compresses to reduce inflammation, numb the area, and relieve acute pain associated with back and sciatica conditions.

Stress Management and Relaxation

Chronic pain is often accompanied by stress, anxiety, and emotional distress, which can exacerbate pain perception and interfere with daily functioning. Implementing stress management and relaxation techniques can help break the cycle of pain and stress.

Stress Reduction Techniques

Mindfulness-Based Stress Reduction: Practice mindfulness-based stress reduction techniques to cultivate resilience, improve coping skills, and reduce stress-related symptoms.

Cognitive-Behavioral Therapy (CBT): Learn cognitive-behavioral techniques to challenge negative thought patterns, manage stress, and promote adaptive coping strategies.

<u>**Relaxation Practices**</u>

Yoga and Tai Chi: Engage in yoga or Tai Chi to promote relaxation, improve flexibility, and reduce muscle tension and pain.

Guided Imagery: Use guided imagery and visualization techniques to create mental images of relaxation and healing, reducing stress and promoting well-being.

Self-Advocacy and Communication

Being an active participant in your healthcare journey involves advocating for your needs, communicating effectively with healthcare providers, and seeking support when needed.

<u>**Communicate Openly**</u>

- ***Express Your Needs:*** Be open and honest with your healthcare providers about your symptoms, concerns, and treatment preferences.

- ***Ask for Clarification:*** If you don't understand something, don't hesitate to ask for clarification or further explanation.

<u>**Seek Support**</u>

- ***Peer Support:*** Connect with others who are living with chronic pain through support groups, online forums, or community organizations. Sharing experiences and coping strategies can provide validation, encouragement, and practical advice.

- ***Professional Support:*** Seek professional support from therapists, counselors, or pain management specialists who can offer guidance, validation, and evidence-based interventions to help you cope with chronic pain.

Lifestyle Modifications

Making positive lifestyle changes can have a significant impact on pain management and overall well-being. By prioritizing self-care and adopting healthy habits, you can optimize your physical and emotional health.

Healthy Eating

Nutrient-Rich Diet: Maintain a balanced diet rich in fruits, vegetables, lean proteins, whole grains, and healthy fats to support overall health and reduce inflammation.

Hydration: Stay hydrated by drinking plenty of water throughout the day to support cellular function, promote joint health, and reduce muscle tension.

Sleep Hygiene

Establish a Routine: Create a consistent sleep schedule by going to bed and waking up at the same time each day to regulate your body's internal clock.

Create a Restful Environment: Make your bedroom conducive to sleep by minimizing noise, light, and distractions, and investing in a comfortable mattress and pillows.

<u>**Stress Reduction**</u>

- ***Mindfulness Practices:*** Incorporate mindfulness practices such as meditation, deep breathing, or yoga into your daily routine to reduce stress, promote relaxation, and improve pain management.
- ***Leisure Activities:*** Engage in enjoyable activities and hobbies that bring you joy and relaxation, whether it's reading, gardening, listening to music, or spending time with loved ones.

<u>**Physical Activity**</u>

- ***Low-Impact Exercises:*** Incorporate regular physical activity into your routine, focusing on low-impact exercises such as walking, swimming, or cycling to improve strength, flexibility, and cardiovascular health without exacerbating pain.
- ***Modify Activities:*** Listen to your body and modify activities as needed to accommodate your pain levels and limitations. Avoid

activities that worsen pain or strain your muscles and joints.

Mind-Body Connection

- ***Practice Gratitude:*** Cultivate a sense of gratitude by focusing on the positive aspects of your life, even in the face of pain and adversity. Keep a gratitude journal or simply take a few moments each day to reflect on the things you're thankful for.
- ***Stay Present:*** Practice mindfulness techniques to stay present and grounded in the moment, rather than dwelling on past regrets or worrying about the future. Mindfulness can help reduce stress and promote emotional well-being.

Goal Setting and Monitoring Progress

Setting realistic goals and tracking your progress can help you stay motivated and focused on your journey toward pain management and improved quality of life.

<u>**Set SMART Goals**</u>

- ***Specific***: Clearly define your goals in terms of what you want to achieve, why it's important, and how you plan to accomplish it.

- ***Measurable***: Establish concrete criteria for measuring your progress and success, such as pain levels, functional abilities, or lifestyle changes.

- ***Achievable***: Set goals that are challenging yet attainable within your current circumstances and resources.

- ***Relevant***: Ensure that your goals align with your values, priorities, and long-term objectives for health and well-being.

- ***Time-Bound:*** Establish a timeframe or deadline for achieving each goal to create a sense of urgency and accountability.

<u>**Track Your Progress**</u>

- ***Keep a Pain Journal:*** Use a pain journal or diary to track your symptoms, pain levels, activities, treatments, and emotional state daily. This can help you identify patterns, triggers, and trends related to your pain.

- ***Monitor Functional Improvements:*** Keep track of changes in your functional abilities, such as mobility, flexibility, and activities of daily living. Celebrate small victories and milestones along the way.

Coping with Setbacks

Living with chronic pain often involves setbacks and challenges along the way. Learning to cope with setbacks effectively can help you maintain resilience and continue moving forward on your journey toward pain management and well-being.

<u>**Practice Self-Compassion**</u>

Be Kind to Yourself: Treat yourself with the same compassion and understanding that you would offer to a friend facing similar challenges. Acknowledge your efforts and progress, even in the face of setbacks.

Avoid Self-Criticism: Refrain from harsh self-judgment or negative self-talk. Instead, focus on learning from setbacks and finding constructive ways to move forward.

<u>**Seek Support**</u>

Reach Out for Help: Don't hesitate to reach out to friends, family members, or healthcare providers for support and encouragement during difficult times. Sharing your experiences and emotions with others can provide comfort and validation.

Join a Support Group: Consider joining a support group for individuals living with chronic pain, either in-person or online. Connecting with others who understand what you're going through can offer valuable insights, empathy, and encouragement.

Conclusion

In the journey of overcoming back and sciatica pain, the empowerment of oneself emerges as a vital aspect. Throughout this guide, we've explored a plethora of strategies, from understanding the intricacies of pain physiology to incorporating holistic approaches for relief.

Empowerment begins with education and understanding. By delving into the complexities of one's condition, individuals can make informed decisions about their health, fostering a sense of control and agency. Armed with knowledge, they can navigate treatment options, communicate effectively with healthcare providers, and advocate for their needs.

Self-care emerges as a cornerstone of long-term pain management. Through a combination of pain management techniques, stress management strategies, and lifestyle modifications, individuals can cultivate resilience and improve their quality of life. From mindfulness practices to physical activity and healthy habits, each self-care strategy contributes to overall well-being and empowerment.

Setting goals and monitoring progress provides a roadmap for success. By setting SMART goals and tracking their journey, individuals can celebrate milestones, stay motivated, and adjust their approach as needed. Along the way, they learn to cope with setbacks with self-compassion and seek support from others who understand their journey.

In the pursuit of empowerment, it's essential to remember that managing chronic pain is a journey, not a destination. Each individual's experience is unique, and there's no one-size-fits-all solution. With dedication, resilience, and a proactive mindset, individuals can reclaim control over their lives, achieve long-term pain management, and cultivate a fulfilling and meaningful existence despite the challenges they face.

By empowering oneself, individuals not only alleviate their suffering but also reclaim their autonomy, resilience, and sense of purpose. As they embrace their journey with courage and determination, they pave the way for a brighter future filled with hope, healing, and possibility.

www.ingramcontent.com/pod-product-compliance
Lightning Source LLC
Chambersburg PA
CBHW051818250726
48659CB00005B/1541